I0422170

INTEGRATED NUTRITIONAL SUPPLEMENTS GUIDE – 1

Digestive Health Supplements

Disclaimer

The purpose of this book is for educational and awareness creation only. It is not intended to be a guide for the treatment of specific medical conditions. Readers having any health issues are encouraged to speak to their primary health care givers for professional assistance. At the time of publishing this book, the information there in was accurate to the best of the author's knowledge. Information is dynamic and so some views and current understanding may change with time.

Murigi Wainaina

Introduction

First off, thank for purchasing this book. It is my sincere hope that it will help you promote your personal health and live a more productive and vibrant life.

This the first book in the Integrated Life series. Under this series we will have various topics that will help us to look at life from a more holistic point of view. The first group in this case is the Integrated Nutritional Supplements Guide. In this guide we have a sub-series of books that include:

- Digestive health supplements.
- Cell care supplements.
- Bone and joints supplements.
- Anti-aging supplements.
- Sexual health supplements.

My suggestion is that you read these books in that sequence as they build from the previous one. However, it is okay to start from any according to your specific needs. This is why this introductory part is available in all the books as I consider it important to the reader. If you have already read it in another book in the series you may opt to skip it and go straight to chapter one.

So, Why an Integrated Nutritional Supplements Guide for You?

An integrated nutritional supplements guide is important because it has a role to play in all the stages of good health management. Optimum health cannot be achieved by the use of just one type of supplement but through a variety. These have to be in the right amount and ratios in relation to other nutrients. Together with a good well balanced nutrition, exercises and a balanced lifestyle, supplements are important in the:

- Preventive stage of health care.
- Supportive role during the curative stage of ill-health.
- Maintenance of a healthy body and mind status.

This guide is about helping you to make informed decisions about the need, the use and the effects of dietary supplementation at any one of the stages above. It is about helping you have meaningful discussions with your health care giver in regards to your health and nutrition needs.

So, how do they help in each of the above three points of your health care? But before we come to that let's answer two fundamental questions: What are nutritional supplements and do I really need them? Let's start with the first and the easy one.

What are Nutritional Supplements?

These are products designed to complement a diet that may be deficient in one or more ways. Many people variously refer to them as food, dietary or health supplements. As the word 'supplement means they play a secondary role in a person's nutritional needs. A good diet is irreplaceable. However, it must be noted that there are many factors that lead to degradation of the foods we eat and hence there is a need to fill these gaps created by deficiencies in our primary nutrition source.

Unlike drugs that generally work on your body to achieve certain desired effect, good dietary supplements work with your body systems by helping them optimize their functions and work naturally as they are supposed to do. In other words they help the body take care of itself and so prevent disease; help fight disease and or help repair and maintain itself.

If the nutritional gaps mentioned above are not covered, over time the effects may manifest in various ways. It may be in form of general ill-health, full disease manifestation or as loss of some body or mental function. Many have attributed their dwindling vitality to age, child birth or other changes in their life. True, these may play a role but the cause could be quietly hidden elsewhere. Later, this guide will detail some of the signs and symptoms that may suggest that you could be in need of fortifying your diet.

So what choices are there for you to consider? The list is long and the various classifications are not few either. There are vitamins, minerals, herbals, proteins, amino acids, probiotics, colloidal minerals and many others. That's not all.

There are also; natural, organic and even artificial supplements. In this series I will help you understand each one of these terms so that choosing and using a nutritional supplement will never be a guessing game again. But before that we need to find out what can lead to poor value in the foods we cat.

Causes of Nutritional Deficiencies.

There are many reasons that can lead to lack of vital nutrients in our bodies. Some of them are:

- Inadequate food intake. This may not be a major issue in the developed countries but it is an important factor in the developing world.

- Poorly balanced food source. One food type may be consumed in large amounts at the expense of the other food types.

- Over-processing of foods. This removes important aspects of the food material that are important to the body's total well-being. So processed foods may have a longer shelf life, may taste better or even look nice but they may turn out to be a precursor to bad health. Since the end of food processing is not likely or even feasible, the option open to many people is to use nutritional supplements or to grow their own foods which may not be practical for many.

- Many agricultural areas have been over-cultivated leading to mineral and other natural soil elements depletion which can lead to mineral deficient crops.

- Lifestyle. Excessive intake of alcohol for example can lead to multiple nutritional related problems. Smoking is also known to affect absorption of vitamin C among others major health issues.

- Age. Advances in age also affect the way nutrients are absorbed into the body.

- Diseases. Certain diseases lead to either excessive or inadequate uptake of nutrients.

These and many other factors have led many people to consider use of nutritional supplements as part of their life.

Nutritional Supplements and Our Environment

Other reasons for considering the use of nutritional supplements have nothing to do with dietary deficiencies but are due to the environment we live in. Our bodies are made in such a way that they can adjust according to the stresses created by our surroundings. In an ideal set-up the body can cope. However, the load of stress factors is getting heavier every day and in some situations we can no longer cope. This has led to chronic states of general un-wellness and disease. These factors include:

- Extensive pollution of the air we breathe.

- Polluted waters we take.

- Increased use of toxic agricultural chemicals whose residues may end up in the foods we eat

- Increased incidence of marine life contamination with heavy metals from industrial waste.

- Increased use of food additives and preservatives which are of no nutritional value to our bodies.

With all these toxic baggage in our bodies the natural systems get overwhelmed. This is when some types of supplements come in handy to help the body get rid of the toxins.

The Nutritional Supplements Journey.

So I invite you to come along with me as we explore the exciting world of nutritional supplements. We will cover:

- Preparing your body for supplements.

- Why everyone may be in need of these products.

- What factors to consider before using them.

- Choosing the right product to suit your age, gender occupation and other factors.

- Frequently asked questions.

- Cell nutrition, vitamins, mineral, herbals, proteins, amino-acids and other types of supplements.

- Precautions and the place of reasonableness in the use of food supplements.

What to Look For when Choosing Nutritional Supplements.

Not knowing what to look for when choosing nutritional supplements has led many people to make important health decision based on hearsay. Sadly, at times the choice is reached due to the hype of zealous sales persons or distributors. That single decision can make the difference between enjoying good health and saving money or losing both money and health.

Knowledge Needed In Choosing Dietary Supplements

With so many nutritional products on the market, choosing nutritional supplements can be a daunting task. For every product, manufacturers and their salespeople make all sorts of claim about the uniqueness and greatness of their product. With this, a person can be overwhelmed and end up making choices that are not based on knowledge. The list below is non-exhaustive but I hope it lives to the aims of the integrated nutritional supplements guide series - helping people make informed decisions about their choice and use of food supplements. Some of the things to look out for and consider are:

Packaging. First impression may be the most important point in choosing nutritional supplements because even the literacy challenged people can fairly judge what they see. How does the packaging strike you? A dubious product may be in a great pack but a good product is unlikely to be in a shoddy pack. Listen to your heart and don't ignore your gut feeling.

Read the label. What are the ingredients? Are there additives to preserve the product? Can the salesperson explain the contents to you in a comprehensive easy to understand manner? On the ingredients list, are there vague listings like 'permitted colors? Questionable ingredients are usually written in hardly legible small print. If part of the label is not readable, think twice before choosing the supplement.

If you are concerned about the amount of sugar in a supplement (and most of us are) look for 'energy' as an ingredient. Many manufacturers label it that way to avoid the word sugar.

Look out also for other common **preservatives** that have been proved unsafe. Examples are sunset yellow and sodium benzoate. Both are suspected carcinogens and may cause hyperactivity disorders.

Ascertain the amount of **ingredients** in the product and compare it with the recommended daily allowance of that nutrient as per the guidelines of your country. Otherwise you may use the USA's FDA standards as a guide.

Investigate and find out the **processing methods** used. Cold processing and molecular distillation are some of the methods that ascertain high quality supplements. However, not all products can be produced this way.

The company. What is the reputation of the company producing and promoting the product? Companies that have been around for a while are more likely to have reliable products.

Product return and refund policy. A company with a fair product return policy is more likely to have good products. It is a sign of confidence with their supplements. Choosing nutritional supplements from such a company can be worth your money.

Do a **Google search** for complaints against the company. Just enter the name of the company followed by the word complaints or scam and there you are with what others have to say. Be cautious however, with colorful positive comments since some of them are made by people with vested interests. A good example is what independent distributors of network companies do in promoting their company's nutritional supplements.

Price may be a consideration factor. Some nutritional supplements are overpriced as a way of compensating the company's distributors. However do not compromise quality for the sake of saving a few coins. The quality of what goes into your body should be above everything else.

Supplement choosing also means knowing some of the possible side effects the supplement may have on your body. This is important if you already have a history of allergy to some foods or other substances.

Get to know the likely interactions with any prescription medicine or other supplements you may be using. Herbal and enzyme supplements should especially be taken cautiously if you are on other medication.

It is good practice to talk to your health-care giver before you start a nutritional supplements program. Even here you must use your judgment since some conventional medical practitioners are not very conversant with nutritional supplement issues and tend to oppose anything they feel is not part of mainstream medicine.

Can any company meet all these requirements? Maybe not; but looking at its profile and products will give you the 'feel' of what you will get.

Other Considerations in Choosing Nutritional Supplements

- **Kosher certificate seal** - accepted by Jewish religious authorities for meeting expected standards.
- **Halal certificate seal** - The Islamic authorities agrees that the product meets their religious standards and expectations for a human consumable product.
- **GMP certification** - does the company boast a certificate of good manufacturing practice company rating or an equivalent depending on your location?
- **DSA**- if the nutritional supplements are sold through independent distributors as in network marketing, is the company a member of your local or international **direct sales association**?
- Any hint of how the company views environmental issues? A company that doesn't care much about our environment may also not care much about your health interests.
- No cruelty against animals seal.
- Council of Responsible Nutrition seal.
- Reputable companies submit their products to independent bodies to analyse and rate them. Look for the label of such companies. An example is the United States Pharmacopeia, USP. Other companies submit their product master file to a pharmaceutical regulating body like USA's FDA. When a company does this, it means they have gone beyond basic requirements for supplements production and are ready to be assessed on the stringent and high scale as pharmaceuticals.
- For the Aloe Vera based supplements, has the supplement been certified by the International Aloe Science Council?
- All or most of these shows to what extent the company goes to to ensure self-regulation and accepts outside scrutiny. The higher the marks a company gets according to your assessment the more likely you are to get a quality product from them.

With this I hope choosing nutritional supplements will be a

much easier affair. For supplements to work better, consider the importance of water and air in your life.

•

The Importance of Water for a Healthy Body.

Without water all body processes will stall and finally die. The best food and the most highly nutritional supplements will be of no use without this vital fluid. So as you get into this nutritional supplements journey, make sure that you take adequate, clean and safe water every day. Consider these reasons for drinking more water as a wider approach to good health:

- Helps to maintain healthy kidneys. Healthy kidneys mean better waste disposal and better health.
- Good and supple skin. The best of skin care products and supplements will not achieve much if the skin is dry and dehydrated.
- Water improves bowel functions.
- It can help you maintain a healthy weight.
- Water will help you maintain the balance of other body fluids.

Fresh Air

This is another factor to consider in the integrated approach to good health. As much as it depends on you, make sure that you are in well ventilated spaces free of polluted air. This may appear impossible but we can all do something about it in our homes where the worst pollution takes place.

CHAPTER 1

DIGESTIVE SUPPLEMENTS

The Gateway to Great Health

Digestive Supplements are probably the most important of all nutritional supplements. Without a smoothly working digestive system, the foods we eat or the supplements we take will not achieve the expected results. In that case, how can we support our digestion system so as to reap more health and vitality?

As always the first step is to have a well-balanced food program. Then our digestive supplements can come in on a supportive role. This way, we will avoid immediate and long-term effects of a poorly working digestion system.

What about nutritional supplements in general? The best of these will be of little to no use if the digestion process has a problem at any of its stages. The use of digestive supplements set the foundation for other nutritional supplements to be efficiently digested, absorbed, assimilated and eliminated from our bodies leaving us enjoying great health.

When Nutritional Supplements Seems not to Work.

One of the main complaints people make about supplements including digestive supplements, is that they never noticed any difference in their overall health even after using them. What could be the cause of this valid complaint? There are many possible reasons but we will only mention a few:

- The length of time the supplements were taken.
- Trustworthiness and quality of the products used.
- Duration of the problem the supplements were expected to relieve.
- Underlying health conditions.

- Poor primary nutrition – food.
- Harmful habits that stress the body. Some of these include; use of tobacco products, excessive use of alcohol and other substance abuse behaviors.

Most importantly, the question is, did the supplements seamlessly go through all the six stages of nutrition? Was the digestion system working well and were the supplements absorbed into the body and assimilated to benefit the user?

The answers to these questions could be the link to a positive experience with nutritional supplements that many people miss. Assuming that everything else is working well then digestive health supplements can provide that connection to better health; not only to the gastrointestinal tract but to the whole body.

Why do we need to Support Our Digestive System?

There are many reasons why our digestive system needs support. The purpose here is to show how digestive health supplements together with an adjustment to dietary and other lifestyle measures can help. We must stress here that some digestive problems must be addressed by your health care provider. Having said that, let's see why digestive health is under attack.

- The foods we eat probably top the list. Like in no other time in the human history, highly refined foods are the norm on many people's tables. This state of fineness slows down the natural gut movement which leads to prolonged retention and impaired elimination (the last stage of nutrition) of gut digestive wastes.
  -
- The refined foods may be profitable to the manufacturers owing to their long shelf-life but they adversely affect the quality and **'shelf-life' of the consumers.**
  -
- Vegetables and Fruits are good for gut health. Sadly, many people do not eat enough of these which further compound the problems created by refined foods.
- The excessive use of saturated fat diets is high and the incidence is increasing in many parts of the world. This can

lead to a sluggish gut and overworked digestive enzymes in addition to other health problems associated with these fats.

- Diseases can be the cause or the result of a bad digestive health status. Any illness that affects the normal operations of the gut's good bacteria will lead to problems with digestion, absorption and elimination stages of nutrition. Needless to say, this will affect our general state of wellness and long-term health.

- Digestive health is also affected by the use of prescription drugs. Antibiotics top the list in this case. These drugs do not differentiate between the normal gut microfloras from the harmful type. They kill all. The use of a relevant digestive supplement comes in handy during or immediately after the use of such an antibiotic. The aim is to maintain or replenish the colony of good bacteria that sustain a good digestive environment. The best digestive supplements in this case are probiotics.
  -

- Heavy intestinal worms infestation grossly affects gut health. Apart from using a conventional de-wormer drug, there is room for a digestive health supplement for the restoration of normal gut activity. Good fiber supplements and certain combined herbal supplements can help in this.
  -

- Low digestive enzyme levels will lead to a sluggish or an incomplete digestion. If this is the case, a digestive health supplement or any other nutritional supplement for that matter may not make any noticeable benefit to the user. This is where a good digestive enzyme supplement come in.

- Finally, for the purpose of our discussion, is a sedentary lifestyle. This could either be due to age, illness or mere laziness. Like any other muscle network in the body, gut muscles benefit from a physically active lifestyle. This can be so through pure gravity effect created by the up and down pressure (imagine someone jogging or jumping the rope) or through demand for more energy following physical exertion which leads to a faster digestion and efficient use of the food or supplements we take.

When all these obstacles have been resolved it will be much easier for nutrients to be useful to our bodies. The full benefits expected when using any other supplement are more likely to be realized

.

The Benefits of Using Digestive Health Supplements.

The following are some of the benefits associated with a healthy digestive system.

- Support in the fight against chronic inflammatory bowel diseases.

- Protection against systemic diseases like diabetes and hypertension.

- Protects against diet related cancers like colon and rectum malignancies.

- They make work easier for digestive organs. For example a digestive supplement like pancreatin makes work easier for the pancreas by providing some of the enzymes like amylase, lipase and protease. These are just a few of the many benefits of using digestive health supplements in addition to a good diet and exercises.

In this book we will examine the exciting world of fiber, probiotics, digestive enzymes, prebiotics and other supplements that make our guts do their job well.

CHAPTER 2

FIBER SUPPLEMENTS

The Trusted Broom for Your Body Systems

Fiber supplements are the ones that do the heavy lifting, so to speak, of clearing the gut of old stools and normalizing emptying and supporting other body functions like your circulation. So in a digestive supplements regime, they may be the logical ones to start with. They do a kind of bush clearing in preparation for other finer details of assisting you achieve greater health.

Maybe you are like many people who have had an occasional delayed bowel emptying for one reason or another. What did you feel when you had that abnormally big gap between motions?

Maybe you experienced headache, nausea, giddiness, some dizziness, dull abdominal pains, heartburn, moodiness and general unhappiness. These are just some of the symptoms that appear when waste is delayed in the bowels. The aim of using fiber foods or fiber supplements is to regulate bowel habits and avoid undue delay between motions. The result is a healthy regular emptying that leaves you feeling refreshed, energized and positive towards life. But what are these nutritional or dietary fibers that we have referred to?

Nutritional Fiber.

The general term used for nutritional or dietary fiber is roughage. These are the plant food parts that a human's system cannot digest. This may be supplied through the diet or through a nutritional supplement containing fiber. There are two main groups of fiber:

1. Soluble fiber

2. Insoluble fiber

Soluble fiber absorbs water to form a viscous gelatinous substance that helps to lubricate stools and hence ease elimination. Insoluble fiber does not change and make the stools bulky which is more friendly to the natural bowel movement, peristalsis. With enough fiber in the diet, the stools are well-formed, fairly bulky but firm and there is a sense of complete emptying of the bowel after each motion. The stools have a diameter of about 1.5 inches. The emptying may be so complete that there is hardly anything on the tissue you use to clean up.

On the other hand, lack of fiber in the diet leads to stagnation of digestive waste in the bowels leading to all types of bad feeling. There is incomplete emptying that, according to some sources, can lead to a gradual stool build up over time. These arrears stools may with time form what may be mistaken for a kind of lower abdomen flab. The residual stools set ground for more serious health concerns both locally on the bowels and the whole body system owing to accumulation of toxins. Among the most serious consequences is cancer of the colon and rectum

Fiber Supplements versus Natural Fiber

Ideally, dietary fiber should be supplied through the normal diet. However, since the advent of commercial food processing and fast food premises, fiber has turned out to be one of the greatest victims of this industrial and commercial development. Most foods have been stripped of this vital component leading to a low grade food product. Some critics have even termed refined foods as *dead or poison foods*. As a result, the West has a higher incidence of bowel related cancers when compared to less industrialized countries where processed foods are not used as much.

Even in developing countries where rural urban migration is an ongoing phenomenon, access to foods rich in fiber is getting more difficult and so the use of highly refined foods is on the rise. In this situation, the only recourse may be to use fiber supplements as part of your wider nutritional supplements program.

Our world is becoming ever so fast-paced that time to think about what is getting into our stomachs is literally not there. As a result, fast food industry mentioned above has become a multimillion dollar industry at the expense of many people's health. Given that our world is forever urging us to be ever faster in whatever we do; many have no time to prepare a meal in the traditional manner. For this group a fiber supplement may save the day and a future.

Let us now briefly have a look at the sources of dietary fiber; the broom that leaves guts and other systems clean and healthy.

Sources of Dietary Fiber are Within Your Reach.

Sources of dietary fiber regardless of whether they are the soluble or insoluble types are from two main groups:
-Plant sources as whole foods.
-Fiber supplements in tablets liquids or capsules forms.

Plant sources of dietary fiber:

Some plant foods can contain both soluble and insoluble fiber. Examples of these **are plums and prunes.** Sources of soluble fiber include **broccoli, carrots, strawberries, bananas and apples.** Other good sources are **potatoes, sweet potatoes and other tubers.** Others are **nuts and psyllium seed husks.**

Soluble fiber undergoes fermentation in the bowels which creates a good media for the guts' naturally occurring non-pathogenic organisms, including good bacteria, to flourish. For that reason, they play an important part in sustaining those organisms. At that point they also become prebiotics which we will discuss in details later in the book. Commercially prepared supplements for this group are available in many shopping malls in the health foods section. They can also be ordered from many online merchants as well as through many reputable network marketing companies.

10 Food Sources of Insoluble Dietary fiber.

There are many sources of insoluble dietary fiber. The list below is by no means an exhaustive one. It only demonstrates that with a little effort many more people can improve on their fiber intake.

1. Whole grain foods
2. Hemp
3. Cauliflowers
4. Avocados
5. Zucchini
6. Unripe bananas
7. Tomatoes
8. Kiwifruits
9. Potato skin
10. Green beans and many others.

Again, this type of fiber is available as a nutritional supplement from many companies.

Fiber Supplements

The main source of these supplements is from plant extracts. As already seen above, there are many types of plant sources. These fiber supplements are usually a combination from different plants and also as a mixture of both soluble and insoluble fiber. Some of the common plants used to make these dietary supplements are: The bran of plants like, wheat, rice barley and oat. Other sources are soy, oranges, apples, peanuts, peaches, to name a few. Combined Fiber supplements are important because different plants have varying fiber characteristics and so the body benefits from them all.

Fiber supplements manufacturers also make the product from **inulins** which are natural **oligosaccharides** in plants like **chicory and Jerusalem artichokes**. Comparatively new in the market are a group called **vegetable gums** which include: **guar gum, acacia gum arabica and acacia Senegal gum.**

From the foregoing, it is obvious that sources of dietary fiber foods are abundant and readily available (we can also add 'affordable') to all of us. Despite this availability many people do not even meet half of their daily requirements. According to The American Dietetic Association, the recommended daily allowance fiber intake for an adult should be 25 to 38 grams. It is important to look for a fiber supplement that will meet your daily requirements. Although we all need fiber supplements from time to time let's see who needs them most.

Who Needs Fiber Supplements?

Fiber supplements may be the only choice for those who are not be in a position to determine the amount of natural fiber in their diets. Examples are.

- Those who are away from home for long like soldiers on active duty.

- Those who eat out most of the time and do not have control over what is sold in food outlets.

- Frequent travelers

- The elderly who may be eating small infrequent meals.

- All those whose diet comprise mostly of refined foods.

- These supplements may also be taken on the advice of a health practitioner as an adjunct to managing a specific health condition.

Whether we are taking fiber supplements because of a specific medical need or we just want to meet our daily requirement needs, the benefits are many. Since sources of dietary fiber are all around us there is really no reason why anybody should be lacking in that respect. Fiber supplements are there to fill nutritional gaps created by unavoidable circumstances or ignorance. Briefly we will discuss the benefits of using these nutritional supplements that are crucial to our total wellbeing.

Short and Long Term Benefits of Using Fiber Supplements.

Benefits of fiber supplements lasting a lifetime? It Sounds like an exaggeration, but is it really? It is not. Within just a few days of taking high fiber diet or supplements, it will take just one complete bowel elimination to notice a difference in your overall feeling. As we will see shortly, other benefits last throughout your life as long as you maintain adequate intake of dietary fiber.

8 Early Benefits of Taking Fiber Supplements

1. Prevention of glucose spikes in the blood. Unlike refined foods a high fiber diet is digested slowly so that energy in form of sugar is released into the blood circulation in sustained manner over a long period. There is no sudden influx of simple sugars into the circulation as it happens with refined foods. Such an influx when repeated for many days harms health in the long-run.

2. Prevention of insulin level spikes. When there is a blood sugar spike, insulin levels correspondingly rise. If this is repeated over a long period, the pancreas can ultimately get exhausted and produce inadequate amounts of insulin. On the other hand the body can become insensitive to the insulin and be unable to control sugar levels in the blood.

3. More energy for longer periods. As we have seen sugar release to the blood is gradual. This provides sustained energy levels.

4. Bowel motions are regularized with better emptying.

5. Prevents food cravings. The bulky nature of fiber leads to a state of fullness that reduces the urge to eat frequently or to consume bigger potions.

6. Prevention of constipation.

7. Fermentation of soluble fiber leads to a good media for the gut's micro-flora to multiply in. This way good bacteria colonies flourish and promotes our health even further.

8. They enhance mineral absorption into the body.

15 Long-term Benefits of Fiber Supplements

Long-term benefits of fiber supplements are a result of accumulated early benefits over a long period of time. On the same note, diseases related to low fiber diet do not occur overnight but come as a result of the body reaching a point where it can no longer cope with the chronic deficiency. Fiber supplements will be important before disease manifestation, once present and even during remission or post-treatment period. Now the benefits:

1. Prevention of chronic constipation and its related problems like; hemorrhoids, anal fissures, and varicose veins.

2. Lowers risk of getting inflammatory bowel diseases (IBD) like ulcerative colitis and Chrohn's disease.

3. Lowers risk of and is good in management of diverticulitis.

4. Is helpful in prevention and management of irritable bowel syndrome (IBS).

5. Lowers risk of getting diabetes.

6. Reduces chances of getting hyperlipidemia.

7. Lowers risk of heart diseases and related complications like stroke and heart failure.

8. By helping maintain normal blood sugar and insulin levels, fiber will ultimately be useful in prevention of vascular diseases like arteriosclerosis.

9. Useful in prevention of hypertension.

10. Important in obesity prevention and may be useful in weight reduction programs.

11. Lowers chances of getting colon or rectum cancers.

12. Fiber diet and fiber supplements have been shown to lower levels of circulating low density lipoproteins (bad cholesterol).

13. The liver is not overloaded with toxins when digestion is smooth and elimination is regular and effective. This leads to an enhanced immunity against recurrent illnesses like gastritis and respiratory infections. Fatigue and other nonspecific complaints are also reduced.

14. Significantly reduces radio-nuclides contamination in the body of nuclear accident victims. This was noted with pectin fiber when used on some of the Chernobyl disaster victims.

15. Finally the benefits of fiber supplements and high fiber foods are that the combined effects of all the above benefits will be easy on the pocket at the personal, national and global levels. You will spend less time and money visiting your doctor. The nation will significantly save resources used in Medicare for conditions related to low fiber diets. Overall the world benefits and can have resources to tackle other health conditions that are not within our immediate control.

Necessary Precautions When Using Fiber Supplements

1. Taking too much fiber can lead to a **deranged acid-base balance** in the body. This is bad for normal physiological functioning of the body.

2. If not taken with enough water, some supplements containing pectin can absorb all the water in the gut leading to serious **constipation**. Note that fiber supplements absorb water many times their own weight.

3. Some fiber supplements have been shown to **interact** with medications for managing **diabetes, depression, epilepsy** and for acute infections that require a **penicillin** to treat. If you are on any medication for these or for any other

condition then you must talk to your health care provider before starting any fiber supplements.

CHAPTER 3

DIGESTIVE HERBAL SUPPLEMENTS.

Digestive herbal supplements have been around in one form or another for the time man and animals have walked the earth. Herbal medicine is one of the oldest, if not the oldest, of all forms of therapies in existence today. Almost 50% of all types of therapeutic drugs today are derived from plants. Many people use herbal supplements to support their digestive system health.

Why Digestive Herbal Supplements?

- There are many reasons why many people use these supplements. Some of these are:
- Promote appetite.
- Help with food digestion through digestive enzymes stimulation.
- Help treat or alleviate acute or chronic digestive system disorders.
- Help prevent or eliminate parasites infestation.
- Promote better bowel movement and elimination.
- As a way of cleansing the gut of old stools and other toxins.

General Grouping of Digestive Herbal Supplements.

This grouping depends on the way the specific herb affects the gut. It must be noted that the effects of these herbs are not confined to the gut alone. They can and they do affect other systems of the body as well.

Demulcents or Mucilages.
Digestive herbal supplements of this nature are sticky mucoid substances that offer a soothing effect to the gut lining. They protect the mucous membranes of the gut against corrosion by gastric acid and other digestive juices. This way, they also reduce gut spasms,

gas and offer protection against toxins and harmful micro-organisms. Examples are supplements derived from or containing licorice, turmeric, ginger, peppermint and fenugreek.

Carminative Herbal Supplements.
The aim of using these digestive herbs is to promote better bowel movement and elimination. This happens through a laxative effect or through increase of stool bulk. They help in relieving constipation. Examples of those with laxative effects are Senna and aloe latex which is derived from the Aloe Vera plant. Herbal products that act by increasing stool bulk are pectin, psyllium seeds, flax seeds, and chia and oat bran. These are common ingredients in many digestive fiber supplements. Supplements in this group must never be used where absolute constipation is suspected. Seek urgent medical attention instead.

Digestive Gut Relaxants.
This group reduces spasms and raised peristalsis. They help reduce diarrhea and excess gas disorders. They are thought to possess effects against microbes, offer antiseptic properties and create a sedative effect to the gut. Examples here are chamomile, cinnamon and lemon balm.

Bitter Digestive Herbs.
The supplements in this group consist of bitter herbs used mostly to increase digestive secretions and hence support better digestion. They are said to reduce gas, food allergies and incidences of indigestion. Examples are barberry root, dandelion, artichoke and gentian.

Anti-inflammatory Digestive Herbs.
These support digestive health in acute or chronic inflammatory conditions of the gut like peptic ulcer disease including bleeding. They can also be helpful in inflammatory degenerative conditions like irritable bowel syndrome and colitis. Turmeric is a good example in this group.

An herb can naturally exhibit more than one property and this grouping here is only for the purpose of highlighting the main properties of particular herbs. The kiwi-fruit and the aloe vera plant are good examples with this quality. As noted above, these herbs can also have good and bad effects in other parts of the body. For example licorice contains glycyrrhizic acid which can lead to raised blood pressure if not removed from the herb. In many cases, herbal products contain more than one herb. Still, others have vitamins and or minerals in them. This makes it important to note and understand all the ingredients in a supplement that you are using.

Presentation of Herbal Digestive Supplements

Herbal supplements are prepared in many ways. They are found as dried products, tablets, liquids, capsules, gels or as powders. They can also be in their natural and unprocessed format. The following are some of the terms commonly used with herbal supplements and remedies:

- **Tea**. This can also be referred to as an infusion. It means adding boiling water to an herb and drinking the product when hot or cold.
- **Decoction**. Product of an herb simmered in boiling water.
- **Tincture**. Product of soaking an herb in alcohol and water.
- **Extract.** Product of removing specific chemicals from an herb followed by evaporation drying. These are then packed as capsules or tablets.

Safety of Digestive Herbal Supplements.

Herbal supplements should generally be taken with caution. Some of them are quite portent and can have undesirable and significant physiological effects on the body. Since many digestive herbal supplements are a mixture of more than one herb, always take time to read the list of ingredients. Then research and find out how each herb or its product affects your health.

If you are on any prescription drugs treatment, or are pregnant, breastfeeding or suffering from a chronic condition, it is important to talk to your health-care giver before taking a herbal supplement. Some herbs interact with certain drugs in ways that can affect the expected results of the drug or produce undesirable side effects. Let's consider one important herb.

Aloe Vera
A Herb of Many Uses.

Aloe Vera herbs have been used for digestive health and other health disorders around the world for millennia. Some sources suggest that the Egyptian queens Cleopatra and Nefertiti used the herb for their cosmetic needs. More recently Mahatma Gandhi is quoted to have said that aloe was among the things that sustained him during his long fasts. Folklore knowledge and scientific research have made the nutritional supplements industry comes up with aloe products that support health on the body as well as in the body.

Some of the benefits associated with aloe vera may not yet have been proved scientifically. However, what is not in dispute is that many people in diverse geographical locations and in different historical periods have used Aloe Vera plant products for their own health and that of their domestic animals. Apart from the nutritional supplements industry, the general home and body care product manufacturers have incorporated aloe as part of the ingredients in soaps, toothpaste and many other products.

Benefits of Aloe Vera.

Supplements from this herb have benefits that involve many body systems. Although in this series we are focusing on the digestive system, to show the extensive benefits of this plant we will include how it positively affects other parts of the body. This to some extent demonstrates how integrative a product's benefits can be on the body for overall wellbeing.

Digestive health.
- It has anti-inflammatory effects and can be helpful in reducing the severity of ulcerative colitis.

- It is supportive in the management of peptic ulcer disease.
- Used in management of constipation.

Skin and topical uses.

- Helpful in the management of moderate burns, skin lesions and bruises.
- Support health in managing herpes genitalis, psoriasis, and dandruff and as a sunscreen. Research findings on this have given mixed results. For this reason an individual may decide to use an aloe product to see whether it will work for any of these conditions that they may be suffering from.
- It has been used in treatment of **radiotherapy** related skin lesions. But again, some researchers have questioned aloe's effectiveness for this.
- Some studies have suggested that Aloe Vera products and supplements may have **anti-skin cancer** properties. This is based on the findings that it tends to raise immunity against this cancer in dogs and cats.
- Promotes healthy hair growth.

Immunity.

- Used as a body systems cleanser.
- Have anti-bacterial and antiviral properties.
- Benefits health in asthma, convulsive disorders, osteoarthritis, immune-suppressive states like HIV.
- Aloe supplements help in alkalinizing the body which is known to promote better health.
- Lowers blood sugar.

Dental health.

- Helps reduce risk or signs and symptoms of gingival sores.
- Lowers harmful lipids in hyperlipidemia.

Nutritional benefits.

- Contains beneficial minerals like calcium, iron, manganese, copper, zinc, magnesium, chromium and sodium.
- Have a wide variety of vitamins including vitamins A, C, E; the vitamin B complex, folic acid and niacin.

- Provides nearly all amino acids that the body needs to function. This includes 8 of which are essential to the body.

Sexual health.

- Promotes good male and female sexual functions. It is said to raise libido.

Cardiovascular health.

- Helps in lowering high blood pressure.
- Reduces blood viscosity.
- Promotes tissue perfusion.

Precautions Interactions and Side Effects.

Aloe Vera supplements and related products are considered generally safe. It is important however to note the following.

Use of the whole plant is not advisable because it contains aloin which has laxative effects. This can cause severe dehydration and related problems like electrolytes imbalance in the body.

People with heart, kidney, liver and bleeding disorders should inform their doctors about their intention to use aloe supplements.

Those on blood thinning drugs, on digoxin, on diabetes treatment, are pregnant or lactating mothers should not use these supplements without consulting their health care giver.

Those going for surgery should stop using aloe supplements two weeks before the operation.

Some of its side effects are diarrhea, visual disturbance, skin rash. A few cases of hepatitis have been reported with its use. This depends on the supplement's degree of purity.

Choosing Aloe Supplements.

Consider the company's reputation, method of production, the mark of quality of the relevant local and international bodies. The best of these marks is the International Aloe Science Council certification mark.

Presentation.

These supplements come mostly as juices but also as capsules and tablets. Topical preparations are in gels, creams, ointments or lotions.

Science may not yet have proved many claims about benefits of Aloe Vera but historical use in diverse geographical locations and subjective reports have made public confidence in it to increase. It has been accepted as a near wonder plant.

CHAPTER 4

PREBIOTICS

In Support of friendly Bacteria Growth.

Prebiotics help the good bacteria in our bodies to multiply and keep us healthy. This term tend to confuse many people into thinking that it means the same thing as probiotics. Nothing is further from the truth. Both however, are important in digestive health and as digestive supplements. A probiotic populates the gut with good bacteria while the former provides the complex sugars that bacteria need as their food to multiply and thrive.

What Are Prebiotics?

These are naturally occurring substances that are described as; "... a selectively fermented ingredient that allows specific changes, both in the composition and/or activity in the gastrointestinal microflora that confers benefits upon host well-being and health." Some of these substances have indigestible food ingredients. This type then qualifies to be called dietary fiber. However, not all fiber foods or supplements qualify to be called prebiotics.

According to Roberfroid, the first scientist to describe them, only two fructooligosaccharides (FOS), naturally occurring plant sweeteners, meet the current definition. They are Oligofructose and inulin. Other scientists have since included galactooligosaccharides (GOS), lactulose and tagatose. Available supplements are mostly based on these oligosaccharides.

To have the best of both words, a combination of these substances and probiotics supplements are now available. Synbiotic is the term used for such a product. A true synbiotic however, is one which can be demonstrated to provide benefits that cannot be achieved by the two products when used separately. The two must have synergistic effects.

Benefits of Prebiotics.

The benefits are many. Some of these are:

1. Improved absorption of minerals like calcium, magnesium and others.

2. Lowering of gut pH which suppresses the proliferation of harmful organisms.

3. Improving immunity status.

4. Reducing risk of getting colon or rectum cancers.

5. Reducing abnormal bowel inflammatory disorders like Chrohn's disease and ulcerative colitis.

6. Reduction of blood pressure in hypertensive patients.

7. Improved bowel movement and quality of emptying which reduces incidences of constipation.

Sources of Prebiotics.

There are two main sources:

1. Natural

2. Synthetic.

Among the natural sources are those of plant origin and those of animal sources.

Plant sources include:
- Raw chicory root
- Raw Jerusalem artichoke
- Raw dandelion greens
- Raw garlic
- Raw leek
- Cooked onions
- Raw onions
- Raw asparagus

- Raw wheat bran
- Cooked whole wheat flour
- Raw bananas
- Other plant sources are kiwi fruits, peas, guinea squash, and agave.

Animal sources include Galactooligosaccharides usually shortened as GOS. This is derived from bovine milk through enzymatic activity on lactose that is found in the milk.

Synthetic sources include:
disaccharides e.g. lactulose
monosaccharides e.g. tagatose

Recently, scientists have started genetically engineering plants for production of inulin. Like many other genetically modified products, the long term effects of such inulin on the user are not known. The prudent thing to do is to know the source of the supplement you are buying so that you can make an informed decision before taking them.

How Much Per Day?

The general agreement is that for ordinary use, an adult needs about 6grams of a prebiotic per day. So if the food source available are bananas which contain only one per cent of the substance, you will need to consume 600grams of the bananas. If you are concerned about calories this might not be an appropriate or even a practical source. If you are also not into raw foods, then the other alternative might be to consider commercially produced supplements. The daily dose may be increased if there is an active problem like any of the inflammatory diseases of the gut.

Choosing a Prebiotic Supplement.

In addition to the general points outlined in the book's beginning about choosing nutritional supplements, consider whether the supplement is of plant, animal or synthetic origin. This is important for vegetarians and some health conscious people who are cautious of using any animal products. Another thing to consider is to confirm whether the product is designed to promote specific good bacteria or it's a general one. This information is usually available on the label.

Precautions and Side Effects of Prebiotics

When first introduced, some people experience flatulence, bloating and abdominal cramps. Starting with small amounts and gradually increasing can help you to get accustomed and finally tolerate them comfortably.

It is common for baby formula manufacturers in some countries to add prebiotics to the baby food. Some countries regulate this and some don't allow it at all. Get to know what is acceptable or not in your country and decide accordingly.

CHAPTER 5

PROBIOTIC SUPPLEMENTS

Probiotic supplements good Bacteria? When many people are first introduced to these supplements they shudder at the thought of consuming live bacteria. In their minds bacteria are organisms to be destroyed with all known methods. What they may not know however, is that the very survival of the human race depends on these microscopic bugs that make a home in our digestive tract. In all cultures, man has been taking one kind or another of foods rich in these organisms.

But just as there are beneficial bacteria in our guts, so are there bad ones. For vibrant health, the helpful bacteria must be available in the right amounts to keep the harmful ones in check. If for some reason the optimal ratio of the good and the bad is disrupted and the good bacteria are suppressed, the bad ones proliferate and disease presents. This is where the supplement comes in. The sole purpose of these products is to augment or replenish the amount of naturally present good gut bacteria.

What Are Probiotics?

This is how the Food and Agriculture Organization, an arm of the United Nations defines them; they are, "...live microorganisms which when administered in adequate amounts confer a health benefit on the host." It is important to understand the difference between the term used here and prebiotics discussed in the preceding chapter.

So as the name suggests, a probiotic ('pro' means 'for' and 'bios' is 'life') supplement is life enhancing. In contrast, an 'antibiotic' has the opposite effect. So on one side probiotics promote the growth of the gut's good microorganisms; while on the other hand, antibiotics kill both the good and the disease causing pathogens. For this reason many health care givers are now including or suggesting the use of these supplements whenever they prescribe antibiotics to their patients.

Types of Organisms Used To Make Probiotics

These include:

Lactobacillus acidophilus of the most which are some of the most commonly used bacteria for production of probiotic supplements. There are many species in this group and they exhibit different characteristics.

Bifidobacteria which are helpful in the management of childhood diarrhea and eczemas among other benefits.

Streptococcus thermophilus
Streptococcus faecius
Saccharomyces bouldii. This is not a bacteria but a yeast.

These organisms are further divided into many subspecies which exhibit different characteristics and health benefits.

Benefits of Probiotic Supplements.
Locally and Systemically

Benefits of probiotic supplements and foods have been confirmed by many studies. Since these organisms offer various benefits and in varying degrees it is good to know the actual organism used and then check some of the benefits associated with it. Some of the benefits are:

Digestive tract health.

Supports health in diarrheal cases. This includes antibiotic induced diarrheal which is a result of antibiotics killing good bacteria together with the bad ones. The rotaviruses are the commonest causes of diarrhea in children. Probiotics have been shown to be supportive during treatment for this type of diarrhea

Ever heard of or even suffered from traveler's diarrhea? It is certainly a bothersome condition that can seriously affect business and fun. Adults who suffer from this do benefit from a probiotic supplement. Lactobacillus acidophilus and saccharomyces bouldii bacteria containing probiotic are useful in these cases

Immune System Support. Allergies of every kind are on the rise due to increasing allergens in our environment and due to the foods we eat. Despite the best efforts by governments and other agencies, our environment is getting more and more polluted. So asthma and eczemas are on the rise. Despite this, some studies have indicated a reduced allergy incidence in children who use probiotic supplements regularly.

Closely related to allergies are inflammatory disorders. These are conditions that follow a disorganized body immune system. A common form of this problem is the Irritable Bowel Syndrome (IBS) and ulcerative colitis. In both these conditions, studies show that probiotics help in reducing the severity of symptoms.

Other benefits of probiotic supplements include improved dental and respiratory health. Usually poor oral health, like dental caries, act as a pool for harmful microorganisms that descend downwards to infect the gastro-intestinal tract, upper and lower respiratory parts. Occasionally, such organisms can affect the heart leading to heart disease.

A large number of people cannot tolerate dairy products. They cannot digest lactose in milk and so they suffer lactose intolerance. Since many probiotics are made with a lactic acid bacteria, the lactose in the dairy product is converted into lactic acid leading to more tolerance.

Peptic ulcerations in adults are a common fact of life to many people. Maybe you have suffered from them or you know someone who has. Either way you know that these stomach ulcers can be debilitating and in some cases have proven fatal following perforation. Together with the standard treatment your doctor may put you on, a good probiotic can help. Some strains of the lactic acid bacteria appear to negatively affect helicobacter pylori, the organism associated with peptic ulcers disease.

Colon cancers have been shown to be related to diets and the overall health of the digestive system. In animal tests probiotics have demonstrated anti-colon cancer cells. It is thought that this effect can also be extended to human beings. To support this thought, users of fermented dairy products have low rates of colon cancer.

Circulatory System Support.

Benefits of probiotic supplements go beyond digestive and immunity support. A significant drop in blood pressure has been established on hypertensive patients put on these supplements.

High Cholesterol levels (the 'bad' type) is also associated with a myriad of health problems including hypertension. Studies have suggested that probiotics can lower circulating cholesterol. The bifidobacterias are particularly good in this respect.

Genito-urinary systems

Probiotics have also been shown to be helpful in some patients with vaginal candidosis. This condition that sometimes follow a course of antibiotic, stress or some diseases like diabetes is quite painful and also an embarrassment to the affected person. Together with other forms of management the supplements help in the management of this as well.

Weight Management.

Other benefits that have been fronted include use in weight

reduction. The data available is however, not enough and many feel that more research needs to be done before this can be advocated as a benefit.

Since many studies have indicated significant benefits of probiotic supplements and foods to our digestive, immunity, heart, circulatory, and genito-urinary system health, it is one of the nutritional supplements everybody should think about. But before using them we need to know how to choose them and precautions to take.

Choosing Probiotic Supplements.

Choosing probiotic supplements need not be difficult. However, all the general factors for choosing nutritional supplements should be considered before taking them as part of your personal health management. Specifically, seek to know the following:

The product should indicate the type of beneficial microorganisms used. That information should include the species and the genus. This is important because different types of these good bacteria exhibit different probiotic effects and benefits.

To the general public, the idea of types, genus and strains might be an uphill task to understand. The most helpful pointer may be the manufacturer's reputation and the label on the product's package indicating that it contains live good bacteria and the approximate number for each.

Choosing probiotic supplements with more than one type of beneficial microorganism is better than a single strain type. This is because as we have already seen various strains have different effects on the host. Such a variety has an overall synergistic benefit on the user.

Liquid, capsule, powder or tablet forms? These are the various ways these products are presented. It's important to know whether the supplement in question needs refrigeration or not. Wrong storage can affect its efficacy. A probiotic supplement that doesn't need refrigeration is more convenient to many users and especially frequent travelers and those who live off the grid. Poor storage can easily kill all the probiotic organisms and all that you would be consuming would be dead bacteria.

When choosing probiotic supplements you need to know how the product is protected against being destroyed by the stomach acids. It must be made in such a way that the maximum number possible of the microorganism used survive the harsh stomach conditions and reach the intestines to deliver their usefulness. This is usually achieved by the manufacturer applying a kind of enteric coating on the supplement that protects the bacteria from the stomach acids. Obviously this is applicable to tablets, capsules and maybe soft gel capsules.

Sources of Probiotics.

Choosing probiotic supplements is also influenced by the origin of the product. The main sources of probiotics are:
1. Probiotic Supplements
2. Dairy products
3. fermented products
4. Genetically engineered probiotics.

Probiotic supplements are perhaps the most used owing to their convenience. They are easy to carry and have specific information about the good bacteria used and the amount. A capsule of quality probiotic contains beneficial bacteria ranging in the billions. To achieve similar levels would mean many servings of say, yoghurt. If you are concerned about body weight issues then a supplement may be what you need. There are both dairy and non-dairy products. So vegetarians can also benefit.

Dairy Probiotics include many preparations at both domestic and commercial levels. Some of these are yoghurt, buttermilk, kefir and yakult.

Fermented products include tempeh, kimchi, sauerkraut and miso.

Genetically modified probiotic organisms are currently available. As with all genetically engineered products, many people are justifiably worried and opposed to this trend of events.

Precautions when using probiotics.

Probiotics supplements are generally safe. However, depending on the type of organism used people with established medical conditions should talk to their health care provider before using them. Those who fall in any of the following groups should be cautious when considering the use of probiotics:

Immuno-suppressed persons.
Those with heart problems.
Those who have undergone some kind of gut resection surgery.

CHAPTER 6

DIGESTIVE ENZYME SUPPLEMENTS.

Digestive enzyme supplements give the digestive system the support it needs in order to fully utilize the food we eat. The right nutrition without enough or no enzymes is of little or no benefit to our bodies. We can compare it to the fuel needed to power an automobile on a good road. Without the fuel, no matter how good the vehicle is and no matter how good the road is, it will just stand there not moving and powerless.

The enzymes start their work right in the mouth, down to the stomach, the small intestines and so on. In good health status this process goes on without much thought of what is happening within our bodies. They quietly and effectively break down the foods into components that can be absorbed into our bodies to keep us alive and enjoying it. A complete enzymes shut-down means that we would be dead in no time.

A sudden shut-down is unlikely but gradual enzymes failure can happen. An operation like pancreactomy will lead to complete cessation of pancreatic enzymes and in that case only enzyme supplementation will help.

Apart from such radical surgery, the gradual enzyme deficiency that many take to be a natural process (and hence do nothing about it) lead to a slow but certain loss in our vitality. This loss may wrongly be attributed to age or other factors. The health conscious will notice the difference and seek to know what could be contributing to this. This search could point to poor digestive enzymes status and after the commencement of the supplement's use, the digestive problems could be solved without doing anything more.

Reasons to Take Digestive Enzyme Supplements.

One of the reasons is when there are signs and symptoms suggesting that the food we eat is not being digested as effectively as it should be. The conclusion then is that probably our bodies are not producing enough digestion enzymes. Some people will reach for conventional symptoms relievers like antacid tablets or liquids while a growing number will think of taking supplements. A few of the signs and symptoms suggestive of inadequate enzymes of digestion are:

1. Abdominal discomfort after taking a fatty meal which was not the case in the past.
2. Inability to enjoy meals that you once enjoyed like meat without some sort of abdominal trouble.
3. Persistent sense of fullness long after taking a meal which some people describe it as 'food just sitting in the stomach.'
4. Heartburn or dyspepsia.
5. Nausea or even vomiting.
6. Growing weakness and loss of vitality and if severe, loss of weight and other disease manifestations.
7. Passing stools with undigested food items.

In themselves this signs and symptoms don't necessarily mean that they can only be caused by digestive enzymes problem. No, other digestion issues can cause similar symptoms. What it means is that digestive enzymes inadequacy is a possibility that should be discussed with your primary healthcare giver. But we also need to know what causes low digestive enzymes.

Causes of Low Digestive Enzymes

Low digestive enzymes can be the cause of chronic abdominal problems like heartburn, bloating and abdominal fullness following an ordinary or even a small meal. In many people's minds the thought of these enzymes being low does not arise and the tendency is to blame other things for their failing health. Let's find out what causes enzyme levels to fall.

1. Age. Some research findings have indicated that digestive enzyme levels fall as we grow old. Many people complain

that they can no longer eat certain foods and enjoy them as they used to do when they were younger. One reason for this could be that the levels of the enzymes involved in the digestion of that particular food has fallen.

2. Some digestive enzymes are provided through fresh fruits and vegetables. Many people do not consume enough of these and so a dietary gap develops.
3. To make the above situation worse, cooking destroys most enzymes.
4. Artificial ripening of fruits is also thought to negatively affect enzyme levels in them.
5. Long distance transportation of fruits and vegetables as well as long stay on the supermarket's shelves lead to low digestive enzymes in them as well as other nutrients in them.
6. With increasing use of genetically modified foods, some people feel that such foods affect digestion and the digestive system.
7. Processed foods are also to blame since vital natural elements have been removed leading to an unnatural food substance.
8. Stress factors like illnesses, extreme temperatures, and chronic fatigue all lead to impaired enzymatic functions which will present as digestive problems.
9. Acquired lifestyle choices like excessive alcohol intake, substance abuse and smoking can also lead to low digestive enzymes production.

Sources of Digestive Enzymes

Low digestive enzymes status can be effectively rectified when we understand where to source our enzymes from. There are three main sources; Plant, animal sources and digestive enzyme supplements.

Plant Sources

1. From fresh plant foods (best raw) like; pawpaws that produce papain, for protein digestion. Avocados have; catalase,

oxidase as well as peroxidase. Others are bananas (contain amylase), pineapples (contain bromelain a protein enzyme), mangos and sprouts which some people consider to be a kind of an elixir of life owing to their abundance in enzymes and nutrients.

2. Generally speaking all fruits and vegetables have varying degrees of useful digestive enzymes. Best results are achieved when they are, taken fresh, are organic and non-GMO.

3. Herbal sources of digestive enzymes include pawpaw leaves and ginger roots that contain zingibain, a protein enzyme which helps in control of auto-immune diseases.

4. Fresh foods. Most of the foods we eat as we have seen are either processed, cooked or if raw not fresh. This in essence makes us eat 'dead foods' which does not give us all the benefits we deserve.

Non-Plant Sources

1. Raw milk contains amylase. Caution should be taken since raw milk is a good media for harmful pathogens to contaminate and multiply. If it is taken for the purpose of the enzymes it must be guaranteed to be from disease-free animals. The highest level of hygiene must be observed from the milking stage to consumption. Raw milk can also be a source of serious communicable diseases like brucellosis.

2. Honey with all its natural ingredients. It must not be processed by heating and again, organic natural sources are the best.

3. The pancreas produces protease, amylase and lipase enzymes. Although they may be present in a fresh and healthy pancreas cooking will destroy them and eating it raw may not be an option for many people.

Nutritional Supplements Sources

Finally, digestive enzymes can be acquired from nutritional supplements. These supplements can either be from the two sources mentioned; animal or plant origin. Some preparations contain both. When choosing a supplement, always make sure of the source in view of allergies to animal products or lifestyle or religious choices. For example vegetarians wouldn't wish to have any digestive supplements of animal source just as a Muslim faithful wouldn't want any of porcine origin.

But what are the specific benefits of using digestive enzymes supplement? Let's find out.

Benefits of Digestive Enzyme Supplements.

The benefits of digestive enzyme supplements are many. They are noted both on the gut and systemically. Improving the quality of the food we take and or supplementing with digestive supplements will help us reap maximum benefits.

Research on the use and benefits of using enzyme supplements is ongoing but some findings suggest that the practice is useful in good health promotion. This is particularly true in the aged, the sick, those whose health has been compromised by wrong food choices and those whose health has been affected by harmful lifestyle choices like substance abuse. The healthy can also benefit by keeping their digestion in tip-top status. Some of the benefits are:

1. Helps the body to fully utilize all nutrients making the user more energetic.
2. Good digestion supplements help in prevention and management of gastritis and peptic ulcers.
3. Helpful in weight management. Enough lipase for example will make more fats to be broken down for energy instead of being stored.
4. All other body systems functions are enhanced as a direct benefit of a good digestive system. For example a good circulation leads to easier waste disposal, healthy liver,

kidneys, brain, skin...all organs. These combined benefits can even lead to a slowed aging process.

5. Leads to less use of antibiotics and other drugs for treatment for palliative management of recurrent abdominal problems due to indigestion.

6. They hasten post-surgery wound healing.

7. They ease work for the body since the natural production of the particular enzyme is not overstretched.

8. Cellulase for example, has been used to successfully manage phytobezoars (an entangled mass of cellulose fiber that can lead to intestinal obstruction.) Use of cellulase can prevent such phytobezoars in the first place.

9. Use of digestive enzymes has been found to be useful in promoting health at the cellular level. This is true of cellulase.

10. Proteolytic systemic enzymes like nattokinase and serrapeptase when taken on an empty stomach help to reduce the thickness, viscosity, of blood. They enhance better blood flow and therefore can be helpful in the overall management of hypertension and prevention of clots forming in the veins like it happens in deep vein thrombosis. This way digestive enzymes can contribute in the prevention of heart attacks and strokes (These two enzyme supplements should however, not be taken together with blood thinning drugs like warfarin, heparin, aspirin and others. Such combinations can lead to serious spontaneous internal or external bleeding.)

11. Nattokinase holds some promise in the management of Alzheimer's disease by breaking down amyloid fibrils toxins which appear with the disease.

12. Alpha galactosidase is an enzyme supplement that has helped people with problems digesting certain foods like beans. When used it minimizes gas and abdominal crumps.

For maximum benefits, nutritional supplements in this group should contain more than one type of digestive supplement. This is because the overall health is not possible with just one type of supplement. Instead the integration of several types gives the body multiple benefits which are a good thing for overall health.

How to Choose a Digestive Enzyme Supplement.

- Go for a supplement with more than one ingredient. A health practitioner may however, prescribe a specific digestive enzyme to address a specific medical need.
- The digestive enzymes supplements in question must be enough to offer the desired benefits. See the amount for each supplement on the label.
- The supplement label must indicate expected benefits and warning signs or side effects.
- Plant sourced digestive enzyme supplements are more versatile in most part of the digestion process.
- On the other hand animal sourced supplements are better when dealing with specific enzymatic needs.

With this guide it is my hope that a nutritional supplement regimen targeting a healthy digestive system is much easier to start and implement. As mentioned early in the book, a healthy digestive system opens the way for all other health products used for various reasons to be assimilated into the body optimally. The end result is a healthy body that shows from the inside out.

The next guide in this series 'Cell-care Supplements' deals with nutritional supplements that promote health at the cellular level. Even with a good digestive system, if the cells are unhealthy or are burdened with toxins, then good health will not be realized.